D0945685

INFLAMMATION NATION

ED WENDLOCHER

Founder and President, Food and Health Research Group, Inc.

Coauthored by Claudia Kreiss

With contributions from
Walter McConnell, M.D., John H. Abel, Ph.D.,
Eugene A. Nau, Ph.D., and Roman Bielski, Ph.D.

WILLARD LIBRARY, BATTLE CREEK, MI 49017

First Edition: 2004

Published by:
Food and Health Research Group, Inc.
Box 768
Wharton, NJ 07885-0768

Copyright 2004.
All rights reserved.

Any reproduction of all or any part of
this publication is prohibited without
prior written permission of the publisher.

ISBN 0-9758835-0-X

www.inflammatoryfoods.com

Cover and text design by Cassandra J. Pappas

WILLARD LIBRARY, BATTLE CREEK, MI 49017

This book is dedicated to my mother,
Catherine Glaab Wendlocher,
with gratitude for her invaluable
encouragement and support.

—ED WENDLOCHER

Contents

Foreword

Consumer and medical media are increasingly reporting the sky-rocketing incidence of inflammatory disease in the United States. In 2002 and 2004, *Time* magazine devoted extensive coverage to the topic. One issue focused on the debilitating disease of arthritis. The other examined the wide-ranging effects of inflammation and linked it to heart attacks, cancer, Alzheimer's, and diabetes.

Inflammation Nation is about my documented discovery of the relationship between common foods in the American diet and inflammation. **That's right—*food and inflammation.*** It grew out of my nearly lifelong struggle with and ultimate victory over a severe condition the medical community calls arthritis. *I call my condition what it is: inflammation and pain caused by sensitivity to toxic food chemicals.*

In *Inflammation Nation* I expose:

- the clear connection between toxic food chemicals and inflammation,
- the liberal use of toxic food chemicals in common foods,
- the lack of testing of these toxic food chemicals, and
- the inadequate labeling of prepared and processed foods that contain toxic food chemicals.

Most important, *Inflammation Nation* offers hope for curbing the inflammation epidemic by identifying immediate actions that you can take to enhance your well-being. *On the basis of breakthrough discoveries made in thorough investigations, I am able to provide an extensive list of specific foods and food ingredients that consistently cause inflammation.* Purging these foods from my kitchen and avoiding them when I go out to eat has allowed me to avoid "the pill trap" and heal. I hope the same will be true for you.

There is a widespread misconception that food has nothing to do with inflammation and pain. *Food has a lot to do with both.* My life, the experience of others, and the food investigations I've been involved with for over two decades prove it.

Ed Wendlocher

Introduction

**A Physician's Perspective on Food, Inflammation,
Ed's Condition, and Arthritis,**
by Walter L. McConnell, M.D.

From 1966 to 1996 I was neighbor and physician to Ed Wend-locher. He was medically diagnosed with arthritis. As his physician, I treated his condition in a manner that was appropriate for that time. The protocol included X rays, drainage of his knees, cortisone shots, blood tests, prescription drugs, monitored over-the-counter drug use, and the possibility of surgery. But I also kept an open mind about how his diet affected his inflammation. *Unlike others who were suffering with the disease and worsened over the years,* **Ed actually experienced an improvement in his condition.** *I believe his success was due mostly to his diligent investigations of food ingredients and his groundbreaking discovery about the link between those ingredients and inflammatory pain.* I wholly support his writing about his experience and success and his efforts to help others.

Because Ed's condition was diagnosed as arthritis, I focus on it here. But current medical research indicates a link between inflammation and several other diseases, including heart disease, cancer, Alzheimer's, diabetes, asthma, stroke, kidney failure, allergy, pancreatitis, fibromyalgia, fibrosis, and anemia. I suspect the list will get longer.

Pain is the most frequent manifestation of the rheumatic diseases. The field of rheumatic diseases encompasses a wide range of diseases and pathological processes, most of which affect joint tissues and thus cause symptoms of arthritis. *Arthritis* literally means joint inflammation: *arth* (joint) plus *itis* (inflammation). *Inflammation is a bodily reaction that causes pain, swelling, redness, and loss of mobility. It is triggered by infectious, mechanical, autoimmune, and/or metabolic factors involving certain foods or the products of the metabolism of foods.*

More simply stated, it is evidence of the body's attempt to heal itself. Ed's condition, and, I suspect, millions of others', was directly related to metabolic factors involving certain foods and the products of the metabolism of foods.

The pathological process most frequently affecting connective tissues in the rheumatic diseases is inflammation. In the past, it was not recognized that inflammation was susceptible to nutritional influences, but it is now clear that fatty-acid derivatives, the prostaglandins, play a key role in the pathogenesis of the inflammatory process, and experimental data have shown that dietary changes can modify the production of prostaglandins during inflammation.

Therapy for arthritis can be very complex, individualized, and related to the type and cause of the arthritis. Traditional therapy has focused on drugs ranging from analgesics, anti-inflammatories (NSAIDS) and steroids, immunosuppressants, and antibiotics. Surgery, including joint replacement, and physical therapy are also common. To date, little attention has been given to diet in traditional therapy; most diet studies and their resultant recommendations have been very shallow, and little consistent success has been achieved through the use of any diet information previously available to the medical profession.

However, in-depth investigations of food ingredients and

arthritis have been completed over the past 20 years, and subsequent research reported by the Massachusetts General Hospital has now indicated a strong relationship between "flare episodes" and the ingestion of certain food ingredients. *The avoidance of these food ingredients and the use of substances to block the effects of these food ingredients hold significant promise in the management of some types of arthritis-related diseases and possibly other inflammation-related diseases.*

1

An End to Life,
or an End to the Suffering?

One day in the mid-1970s I lay in excruciating pain and despair thinking I would not live to the end of the decade. The arthritis I had been diagnosed with and battling since I was 10, which at best hobbled me and at worst left me bedridden for days, looked as if it had finally defeated me. Many persons in the medical community I had met, who refused then to believe that diet had anything to do with the inflammation and pain I lived with, were telling me that my liver might soon fail, having been pummeled by heavy medication for four decades. My wife had left me, weary of living with an angry, disabled man. I actually began to hope I would die and be liberated from my disastrous, pain-filled life.

*Then something shifted in my thinking. I resolved that I wanted to live, that I wanted to be healthy, and that if I truly believed what in my heart I knew to be true, **that diet affected my pain,** then it was going to be up to me to do something about it.*

1

For the past decade I have watched what I eat and have been practically pain-free. I am in the best shape I've been in all my life. I care for a half-acre garden, cut and split cords of wood for my wood stove, and can even jog. I am remarried, to a wonderful woman, and my outlook is positive.

Being stuck in a cycle of pain can be very depressing. I know others of all ages who have coped with the emotional strain caused by physical pain. I did. As a child, I was affected by my arthritis in everything I did. With swollen knees wrapped in bandages, I often couldn't play with the other kids or participate in team sports. I routinely had to have my knees drained and get cortisone shots. In high school I had to take the freight elevator, as I was unable to walk up or down the stairs. The college that accepted me was on a mountain. Getting around campus was at times nearly impossible. I disguised my disability as best I could and never spoke of it, fearing I'd be seen as not normal. I'm sure this compounded my emotional pain, but it also helped build a strong will.

People in pain sometimes report that their discomfort inexplicably recedes and they experience a period of relief. I was lucky for a short while after I graduated from college. In hindsight, I realize that my diet improved as my income rose. I no longer had the daily habit of eating my favorite sandwich, bologna with ketchup, which I'd eaten since childhood and now know was, for me, highly toxic. I began to lose excess weight. My confidence grew. I dated and eventually fell in love with a beautiful woman, whom I married. My life seemed on track for the first time. But eventually the pain returned, and I spiraled down again.

During my 30s and 40s I was often unable to get out of bed except to crawl to the bathroom. When I was able to get up, it was usually with the aid of crutches or a cane. (The good news is that I learned that, *most* times, drivers stop for people on crutches trying to cross the street.) My doctors diagnosed my condition as rheumatoid arthritis, mostly of my knees and hips. X rays showed arthritic ridges and valleys between my knee bones and my kneecaps. I took daily heavy doses of aspirin (up to 20 pills) and prescription drugs and continued to have my knees drained regularly and injected with cortisone so that I could keep going.

Over the years I noticed that the inflammation, pain, swelling, and stiffness were worse after I had eaten spicy foods but better after I'd been too sick to eat for several days. Fortunately for me, Dr. McConnell was open-minded about the issue and encouraged me to investigate how foods might be affecting my pain.

The Journey Back to Health

After hitting bottom in the early '70s, I began my journey back to health. Then, when my mother fell to her death, stumbling down the cellar stairs because her twisted, arthritic, clumplike feet were unstable, my determination to find a solution to my problem became even greater. Along my journey I met many extraordinary people, including Dr. Norman Childers and Dr. Ambrose Zitnak, two individuals who conducted pioneering research in food toxicity. Talking with them facilitated a great unburdening in me, as they confirmed my belief that food could cause inflammation and pain. I am grateful for their friendship and encouragement.

It has also been very satisfying to meet a wonderful doctor who did not believe what I said about the side effects of some foods but who changed his mind when some of his patients improved after avoiding those foods. He is Leo Galland, M.D., F.A.C.D., F.A.C.N., and we remain friends today. But my greatest satisfaction, now that I have saved my own life—*and I believe I would not be here today if I had followed the guidance of the traditional medical system*—is in helping others. Which brings me back to you, the reader, to whom I wish to be of service. Seeing others find a solution to the problem of their pain is that for which I am most grateful.

Thankfully, our discoveries have also enabled me to help my family, including my daughter Gretchen and my son Edwin Jr., who are predisposed to the condition. Both adhere to the dietary recommendations. For Gretchen, who is more adversely affected, it means being able to continue to pursue her passion for dance and dance instruction. Unfortunately, my grandchildren, 10-year-old Edwin III and four-year-old Dylan, are also showing signs of sensitivity: a red flush on their faces when they eat a "problem" food. Fortunately, our family has the knowledge that can help them. You too can have that knowledge.

In 1979 I founded a food research group consisting of physicians, scientists, and medical graduate students and worked with family, friends, and hundreds of people who wanted to know more about the causes of inflammation, pain, swelling, and stiffness.

The core research group has now completed the first ever, 20-year-long, thorough and accurate investigations of more than 1,000 foods and food ingredients.

Our research clearly showed a strong relationship between flare episodes of inflammation, pain, swelling, and stiffness and the ingestion of certain food ingredients.

The solution to my problem lay in changing my diet. Today I successfully manage my inflammation and pain by very conscientiously avoiding problem foods and food ingredients. I regularly take some aspirin, which is also for the health of my heart, and health products specially formulated to counteract the effects of the problem food ingredients when I inadvertently eat some.

Inflammation Nation is about my journey, but it offers powerful, detailed information that may help you eliminate, significantly reduce, or, at the very least, better manage your inflammation, pain, swelling, and stiffness. It discusses the research group's independent investigations and includes information about research conducted at Harvard Medical School and reported by the Massachusetts General Hospital. It tells of the experiences of others who have found relief by changing their diet, and, *unlike any other book, it provides a detailed list of potentially inflammatory foods, as well as foods found not to be bothersome.* Awareness of and change in diet (and there are plenty of great foods to eat) have already helped hundreds of people, from two to 82 years of age. I sincerely hope it will help you too!

2

Identifying the Problem:
A Turning Point in Food Investigations
Leads to a Major Breakthrough

I am an environmental health and safety (OSHA) engineer (B.S., Lehigh University, Bethlehem, Pennsylvania) and consultant. My career has made me very familiar with asbestos, formaldehyde, vinyl chloride, and toluene and the devastating effects these and other chemicals can have on the human body. To me it was common sense that food "chemicals," naturally occurring toxins, might also affect the body. In 1981, two years after founding the food and health research group, I launched the first of four investigations into food and food ingredients. It lasted nearly a decade.

My research also included 25-, seven-, and 100-person studies. Information about the 25- and seven-person studies, conducted by the Food and Health Research Group, Inc., follows. Information about the 100-person study, conducted by the Arthritis Help

Centers, which involved the use of supplements, is in the back of the book.

I lead you through all the investigations and studies because I want to share how serious I was about rooting out the cause of my problem and how I arrived at the solution.

Launching Food Investigations

To get the first food investigation under way, I developed a detailed list of foods that I suspected might cause inflammation, pain, and stiffness. My resources were my own experiences with food plus food and nutrition reference guides to the basic plant and animal families of foods usually eaten in the United States. With this list a food investigation was begun that included hundreds of foods. With a small group of dedicated volunteers, the food research group began to systematically investigate each food to see whether it caused inflammation, pain, swelling, or stiffness.

Volunteers were assigned 10 foods for evaluation. While eating a simple diet that included only the foods already known not to cause inflammation, pain, and stiffness, each volunteer would then eat a sample of the food to be investigated and report whether he or she thought it caused a reaction. Over the following years this activity was repeated over and over with additional volunteers who suffered from different types of arthritis, until each food had been carefully investigated.

In 1984, the investigations were revised so that they would be more exacting, and careful attention was paid to what foods were being eaten in a meal. For example, roast chicken and a soft drink became white-meat chicken, corn oil, black pepper, dairy butter, table salt, onion, and natural lemon/lime-flavored soda. The investigations were continued until each food and food ingredient had again been carefully and reliably investigated. The foods or food ingredients found to cause inflammation, pain, swelling, and stiffness during these investigations were then each reassigned to groups of new volunteers to verify.

By 1989, clear patterns had begun to appear in the mostly inconsistent results, and foods or food ingredients were ranked generally as:

1. clearly and repeatedly appearing to cause inflammation, pain, swelling and stiffness,
2. clearly and repeatedly appearing NOT to cause inflammation, pain, swelling, and stiffness, and
3. producing results mixed or unclear.

The foods in group 3 (results mixed or unclear) were reinvestigated for an even more exact review of what the volunteers were eating. We contacted food companies to identify food ingredients, *particularly the flavor enhancers and preservatives listed on their labels in general terms, such as "flavorings," "colorings," or "spices."* We studied the U.S. government's FDA (Food and Drug Administration) food ingredient and food labeling laws and regulations to learn more about food names and food contents.

A Turning Point Leads to Significant Breakthroughs

Our obtaining greater accuracy about foods and food ingredients from food manufacturers and our becoming knowledgeable about FDA food ingredient and food labeling laws were major turning points in our investigations.

We discovered two crucial and very surprising facts:

1. ***Not all food ingredients are required to be listed on the labels of some foods.***

    For example, paprika in red wine vinegar or in cheese does not have to be listed on the product label.

2. Many food ingredients are allowed by law to be listed only as flavorings or colorings.

For example, red pepper added to cola and paprika in mayonnaise may be listed as natural flavorings.

These facts may be common knowledge among food industry professionals and government regulators, but most people do not know about them. We didn't.

So, we amended the food investigations as necessary, so that each food ingredient in a food in the "results mixed or unclear" group (3) was being investigated, rather than the total food. *This detailed approach led to another breakthrough and appeared to improve dramatically the consistency of the results.* **Once all ingredients had been accurately identified, confusion was reduced and clear, consistent results produced.**

By 1990, many foods had been added to the list, and a master list of more than 1,000 foods and food ingredients was developed, tested, and retested. Three new groups of foods emerged:

1. **foods that clearly appeared to cause inflammation, pain, swelling, and stiffness;**
2. **foods that clearly appeared NOT to cause inflammation, pain, swelling, and stiffness; and**
3. **foods that appeared NOT to cause inflammation, pain, swelling, and stiffness by themselves *but that are often served with other ingredients that do.***

It's important to note that I am referring here not to the familiar, instant pain often felt as these ingredients are eaten and that affects the mouth and upper digestive system *but rather to delayed inflammation, pain, swelling, and stiffness felt one to three days later in the muscles and joints of the body,* which is usually when the symptoms appear.

- After nearly a decade of research, our findings concluded that the major food or food ingredient found to cause inflammation, pain, swelling, and stiffness is the "hot" chili pepper in any form.
- We also discovered that the "hot" chili pepper may be hidden in food and labeled as a spice, a spice extract, a flavoring, a natural flavoring, a seasoning, a coloring, or a preservative. It may also be omitted from a food label.
- The "hot" chili pepper, in any form, is in hundreds of foods Americans eat every day.

The "hot" chili pepper, which is actually a fruit (although the U.S. Food and Drug Administration classifies it as a spice), has captivated people's imagination for centuries. It is a colorful part of folklore, inspires culinary artistry, and sates many an appetite for a zesty food. The chili pepper is also noted for its beneficial medicinal properties, including a high vitamin C content and the ability to raise endorphin levels. I am not disputing its benefits. *However, the "hot" chili pepper contains capsaicin, a natural toxic food chemical that can have profound negative effects and which I discuss at length in this book.*

I unequivocally believe that many people can eat the "hot" chili pepper, in any of its forms, and not be adversely affected. The digestive systems of some persons apparently can efficiently block its effects, and few or no symptoms occur; others cannot. Some persons have a sensitivity at birth, while others seem to become sensitive with age. *But for those who suffer inflammation, pain, swelling, and stiffness, the chemistry of the "hot" chili pepper could cause physical problems, or make problems worse, as our studies indicate.*

If you're thinking, "I don't eat chili peppers," think again, because you probably do. When I tell people about the adverse effects of the "hot" chili pepper, nearly 100 percent say they eat very little or none at all. But when they learn the startling fact that it is an ingredient often hidden in hundreds of common foods we eat every day, including the broth in canned tuna fish, they reconsider.

Please note that I am NOT advocating that anyone managing his or her inflammation, pain, swelling, and stiffness with over-the-counter drugs or prescription medicine abandon those drugs. I AM suggesting that those persons develop a keen awareness of diet, modifying it as necessary and noting the positive results. As always, please talk with your doctor before making any changes in your diet or lifestyle.

CHAPTER TWO RECAP

- Not all food ingredients are required to be listed on a food product label.

- Many food ingredients are allowed by law to be listed only as flavorings or colorings.

- The Food and Health Research Group's investigations demonstrated that the food and food ingredient that consistently causes inflammation, pain, and stiffness is the "hot" chili pepper in any form.

- The "hot" chili pepper may be hidden in a food and labeled as a spice, a spice extract, a flavoring, a natural flavoring, a seasoning, a coloring, or a preservative.

- Accurate identification of all ingredients in foods investigated produced clear, consistent results about the connection between food and inflammation.

- The "hot" chili pepper contains capsaicin, a natural toxic food chemical.

- Ingestion of the "hot" chili pepper in any form can lead to inflammation, pain, swelling, and stiffness one to three days later in the muscles and joints of the body of some persons.

- Nearly 100 percent of the people who learn from me about the adverse effects of the "hot" chili pepper but believe they eat little or none of it are shocked to discover how abundant it really is in their diet.

3

Understanding Inflammation— Medical and Personal Points of View

As Dr. McConnell explained, inflammation is triggered by infectious, mechanical, autoimmune, and/or metabolic factors involving certain foods or the products of the metabolism of foods. The body's reactions are manifested as pain, swelling, redness, and loss of mobility.

The highly complex inflammatory response is of great interest to the medical community, which currently spends billions of dollars researching it and developing medications to manage it, as well as to the individuals who are suffering with it. Enter the term *inflammation* or *inflammatory disease* in an Internet search engine, and you're likely to receive well over 2,000,000 results—a good indication of how much a part of our consciousness the subject has become.

In February 2004, *Time* magazine ran a revelatory cover story about inflammation. The headline read: "THE SECRET KILLER— The surprising link between INFLAMMATION and HEART

13

ATTACKS, CANCER, ALZHEIMER'S and other diseases. What you can do to fight it."

The reporting, which appears on pages 38 through 46 of the magazine, includes a clear, simplified description and illustration of the body's inflammatory response to a wound. The editors cite their sources for this information as Dr. Moses Rodriguez, Mayo Clinic; Dr. Gailen Marshall, University of Texas–Houston; and *Scientific American*, May 2002.

As the *Time* article notes, the inflammatory response is a very complex and not entirely understood chemical reaction. Essentially, it is part of a healing process—a kind of counterattack when the body thinks it's under attack, whereby blood and immune cells move to an injured area to control damage and promote healing.

According to the article, "researchers believe that the same system that causes inflammation around a wound can—when the response becomes chronic—play an important role in a broad range of illnesses," such as heart attacks, heart disease, arthritis, diabetes, Alzheimer's, and cancer.

I understand my own inflammatory response as a metabolic experience and have made the following connection between my diet, which contained the "hot" chili pepper (as a spice, a spice extract, a natural seasoning, or a coloring), and the inflammatory response in my body:

- The "hot" chili pepper, in any form (spice extract, natural seasoning, or coloring), which contains capsaicin, was ingested and entered my bloodstream.
- Capsaicin, a natural toxic food chemical, attached itself to the chili pepper cell receptor, technically called TRVP1, and damaged these target cells. (See chapter 10 for information about p38 and TRVPI.)
- My immune system responded and attacked the damaged cells in an attempt to manage the perceived "invasion."

- Damaged tissue and cells released factors, such as prostaglandins and nerve growth factor, that promoted inflammation.
- Capsaicin also bound to TRVP1 on my nerve cells and induced pain.
- The factors released after prolonged inflammation and extensive tissue damage increased the number of TRVP1 receptors on my pain nerve fibers, making them hypersensitive to capsaicin.
- My joints became supersensitive to touch, heat, and capsaicin, causing excruciating pain.
- The invasion persisted for years as I unwittingly ate foods that contained the "hot" chili pepper hidden in foods.
- I became disabled with intense inflammation that was diagnosed as arthritis.

It is important that the *Time* article asks what happens if inflammatory fires flare up for prolonged periods or simply don't die down. Doctors and researchers say that disabling symptoms and tissue damage may result. According to the *Time* article, the damage may be permanent. My answer to the question is that there is lots of pain and suffering and, as in my case, debilitating arthritis.

In my opinion, the inflammation response in my body was not able to recede until I stopped eating foods and food ingredients that contained the "hot" chili pepper (with capsaicin). When I stopped eating problem foods and food ingredients, I believe, the cells in my body were no longer being damaged by the "hot" chili pepper (with capsaicin) and my body was relieved of the need to respond to the "injury" with an inflammatory response. The inflammatory fires were extinguished, my body stabilized, and I returned to health. I think the same process might occur in others.

Last, another thing known about inflammation is that, as Dr. McConnell notes in his introduction, the prostaglandins play a key role in the pathogenesis of the inflammatory process. Prostaglandins are chemical mediators that regulate cell functions.

Some prostaglandins intensify and increase the inflammatory response, while others reduce it, acting as anti-inflammatories. Prostaglandins that are inflammatory are produced from a fatty acid called arachidonic acid. They are commonly found in animal foods (especially red meat). The more animal fats consumed, the more arachidonic acid is produced in the cell membranes and blood and the higher the level of inflammatory chemicals. Dietary changes—specifically, a reduction in the consumption of animal fats—can modify the production of prostaglandins.

CHAPTER THREE RECAP

- Inflammation is a complex chemical reaction initiated by the body as it attempts to heal itself. It manifests as pain, swelling, warmth, and redness.

- Researchers believe that the same system that causes inflammation around a wound can play an important role in a broad range of illnesses.

- Current medical research links inflammation to heart attacks, heart disease, Alzheimer's, diabetes, cancer, and arthritis.

- My experience links the ingestion of the "hot" chili pepper in any form (spice, natural flavoring, coloring, and so on) to my inflammation.

- When the "hot" chili pepper in any form (spice, natural flavorings, colorings, and so on) was eliminated from my diet, the inflammatory fires in my body were extinguished and I healed.

4

Studies Participants Demonstrate Link Between Problem Foods and Inflammation and Pain

I believed I wasn't the only one suffering with inflammation and pain as the result of eating problem foods, so in 1994, following the decade-long food investigations, I organized a 25-person study, which was conducted by Professor John H. Abel, Ph.D., at Lehigh University, in Bethlehem, Pennsylvania. The purpose of the study was to evaluate whether persons diagnosed with arthritis and presenting inflammation, pain, and stiffness could benefit by not eating the foods found to trigger a reaction. Twenty-five volunteers with different types and varying degrees of severity of arthritis were requested to avoid conscientiously during a six-week period the foods found to cause pain, swelling, and stiffness. Each was requested to record his or her ranking of pain, swelling, and stiffness at the beginning of the six-week study and at its end.

The result: Two reported remarkable relief, 17 reported major relief, and six reported some relief of pain, swelling, and stiffness.

Later in 1994, Eugene A. Nau, Ph.D., an immunologist and visiting scientist working with Professor Abel at Lehigh University, led a dramatic, seven-person study. The purpose of that study was to evaluate whether persons with arthritis who had been avoiding the problem foods would experience a worsening of inflammation, pain, and stiffness after eating a meal containing four to five of the foods already found to cause problems. Seven volunteers with different types and levels of severity of arthritis donated a blood sample for analysis prior to the meal, were treated to a meal containing foods found to cause inflammation, pain, swelling, and stiffness, and donated a second blood sample for analysis following the meal.

The result: Two reported very severe pain, swelling, and stiffness and five reported some additional pain, swelling, and stiffness two to three days following the meal.

Analyses of blood samples showed a significant rise in the inflammation levels measured in all seven persons for blood samples taken three days after the meal compared with those taken before the meal.

CHAPTER FOUR RECAP

- In a 25-person study in which participants were asked to avoid "trigger" foods, every individual found relief from his or her inflammation and pain.

- In a seven-person study in which participants who had avoided "trigger" foods were asked to eat a meal containing problem foods, everyone reported pain, swelling, and stiffness two to three days after the meal.

- In the seven-person study, participants' blood samples taken three days after the meal containing "trigger" foods showed a significant rise in inflammation levels.

5

A Very Brief Introduction to Spices and the "Discovery" of the Chili Pepper Fruit

W hat is it about the "hot" chili pepper that is problematic to some people? The answer is complicated, so I begin with a brief introduction to spices and the "discovery" of the chili pepper fruit and follow that with information about natural toxins in plants.

Pictorial and written records indicate that we began using spices for flavoring as early as 5000 BC. In 525 BC the Greek philosopher Pythagoras records medical notes on human sensitivities to some foods. In 90 BC the Christian prophet John of Ephesus writes (Revelation 18:11–13) that the use of spices is one of the excesses that will bring about the fall of Babylon. In 40 BC Marc Antony's wife, Fulvia, describes a lavish banquet of spicy dishes originating in the Far East. Many books have been written about the "spice routes" across Europe, the Middle East, and the Far East and about the significant impact spices have had on world history. Many world explorations during the last millennium were driven at least in part by the quest for spices. In the past, spices were a commodity much sought after and the most expensive item in the pantry of foods enjoyed by royalty and the very rich.

It wasn't until 1492, when Christopher Columbus "discovered" the new capsicum pepper fruit (the "hot" chili pepper) in the West Indies, that spices began to be more reasonably priced and could be afforded by people of modest means. These new, less expensive, tastier varieties soon spread around the world, and they began to be used widely to preserve meats and even to disguise the bad smell and taste of spoiled meats on ships traveling to all parts of the globe. Columbus himself loved the new capsicum (in the form of cayenne pepper) varieties, ate them regularly, suffered from arthritis, and died in 1506, a deformed cripple no longer able to stand or walk.

Numerous spicy dishes became very popular in America during the 1700s and 1800s as the "hot" chili pepper fruit spices were added to many foods existing at the time and combined with the newly discovered tomato. That trend continues today. The "hot" chili pepper can be found in hundreds of foods in nearly every country around the world. It is estimated that, worldwide, people consume tens of millions of tons of the "hot" chili pepper spice annually.

CHAPTER FIVE RECAP

- **Many world explorations during the last millennium were driven at least in part by the quest for spices.**

- **After Christopher Columbus "discovered" the new capsicum pepper fruit (the "hot" chili pepper) in the West Indies, spices began to be more reasonably priced and could be afforded by people of modest means.**

- Columbus himself loved the new capsicum (in the form of cayenne pepper) varieties, ate them regularly, suffered from arthritis, and died in 1506, a deformed cripple no longer able to stand or walk.

- It is estimated that, worldwide, people consume tens of millions of tons of the "hot" chili pepper spice annually.

6

Natural Food Toxins, the Link to Pain, and How the FDA and the EPA Are Involved

Most people have the good sense not to eat unidentified plants in the wild. They naturally suspect that whatever is growing in a forest or a field might be poisonous. While some plants that grow in uncultivated land are safe to eat, many are poisonous and produce toxins that can cause pain, swelling, stiffness, and even death.

Few of us are aware, however, that nearly *all* plants produce some amounts of natural toxins called glycoalkaloids or simply alkaloids. These organic, nitrogen-containing substances are part of a plant's natural defense system and protect it from animal predators. Many alkaloids possess potent pharmacological effects and are used medicinally to fight the symptoms of disease, in a beneficial application of natural toxins. You'll recognize the names of a few of the alkaloids: cocaine, strychnine, nicotine, caffeine, morphine, mescaline, methamphetamine, pilocarpine, piperine, atropine, ephedrine, and tryptamine.

The "hot" chili pepper alkaloid is called capsaicinoid and is found in many foods.

Contrary to popular belief, the Food and Drug Administration does not test all food ingredients for their health effects on humans. In addition, the laws of the Food and Drug Administration specifically state that the FDA deems it impractical to list all food ingredients commonly used in foods. In particular, most food flavorings, natural flavorings, seasonings, spices, and spice extracts commonly used in foods prior to the promulgation of the FDA food laws were not required to be proven safe once those laws became effective.

The Food and Drug Administration and the U.S. Department of Agriculture work to control many of the toxins in our foods, but their emphasis has been on toxicity in humans (does the food cause serious impairment or death?) or on carcinogenicity (does the food cause cancer?). These agencies allow "permissible amounts" of toxins to be present in foods as long as the amount is assumed not to cause serious impairment, cancer, or death.

The Food and Drug Administration laws also make it difficult to identify and test ingredients in a food. *Ingredients of many foods need to be shown on the label only as flavorings, colorings, natural flavorings, seasonings, spices, or spice extracts, without any further identification. Some ingredients in food need not be identified on the label at all.*

At the time of this writing, the Food Allergen Labeling and Consumer Protection Acts (S. 741) became law. Effective January 1, 2006, the legislation requires food manufacturers to clearly label eight problematic ingredients: milk, eggs, fish, crustacean shellfish, tree nuts, peanuts, wheat, and soybeans. The bill also requires food ingredient statements to identify food allergens used in spices, natural or artificial flavorings, and additives. This important legislation is a significant achievement, but it does not solve the problem for people who are sensitive to the adverse affects of the "hot" chili pepper.

It is difficult for most people to know exactly what is in the foods they eat, much less accurately know what their effects are on health. Following the early food investigations, we researched the problem foods (those containing the "hot" chili pepper used as a flavoring, coloring, natural flavoring, seasoning, spice, or spice extract) and found that *they contain capsaicin, the alkaloid that puts the "hot" in the "hot" chili pepper.*

Capsaicin is listed in scientific reference books as a poisonous, toxic chemical with an LD50 value that should draw concern. LD50 values are scientific measures of animal toxicity of a substance, indicating the dosage at which at least 50 percent of the test animals fed the substance died. Comparing the LD50 value of capsaicin with the LD50 value of nicotine in the tobacco plant (which is a "cousin" to the "hot" chili pepper), you'll find that capsaicin is in the same league as the dangerous toxin nicotine in cigarette smoke.

In 1962 the Environmental Protection Agency approved capsaicin as a pesticide for fruits, vegetables, grains, flowers, and ornamental trees because minute quantities were found to kill pests effectively through cardio-respiratory seizure. Capsaicin was re-certified by the EPA in 1994 and is still used today as a deadly pesticide.

The EPA describes the effects on human health of capsaicin as *"negligible due to the long history of use by humans as a food additive/component without any indications of deleterious health effects."* In addition, the EPA states, *"[T]he agency has waived requirement for toxicological data due to its presence in the human diet."*

What I understand by the above statements, in information available to the public as of this writing, is that the Environmental Protection Agency has approved capsaicin for use as a pesticide and has NOT tested capsaicin for its health effects on humans, nor does the agency believe there is a need to test it to find out whether it is harmful to humans. Leadership at the EPA and at the FDA might be interested to learn of the following, presented by Roman Bielski, Ph.D., on the harmful toxic alkaloids found in many foods, including capsaicin:

"Humans are susceptible to poisoning by the plant toxic alkaloids. Symptoms of this poisoning are a bitter taste and a burning sensation in the mouth and throat, gastrointestinal tract irritation, inflamed intestinal mucosa, ulceration, hemorrhage, stomach pains, diarrhea, apathy, drowsiness, salivation, labored breathing, trembling, ataxia, muscle weakness, paralysis, loss of consciousness, and death due to cardio-respiratory paralysis."

In most cases the fruits, seeds, leaves, stalks, roots, and other parts of plants selected to be safe for human consumption have only very small amounts of harmful toxins in them. But because each of us metabolizes food differently, I think it's prudent to say that we would be better served if we were aware of the natural toxins in the foods we eat, especially when they are used in prepared foods and not included on the ingredients label.

I think it's also time for the EPA to reassess a decades-old decision and test capsaicin for its effects on human health. I also think it is time for the FDA to require the clear, accurate listing of capsaicin in food.

CHAPTER SIX RECAP

- **Plants contain natural chemicals that are toxic. These are called alkaloids or glycoalkaloids and have effects both beneficial and harmful on humans. The "hot" chili pepper alkaloid is capsaicinoid.**

- **Capsaicin is listed in scientific reference books as a poisonous, toxic chemical with an LD50 value that should draw concern. Its**

LD50 value is comparable to the LD50 value of the dangerous toxin nicotine in cigarette smoke.

- The EPA has NOT tested capsaicin to find out whether it is harmful to humans and does not believe there is a need to conduct such testing.

- The EPA has approved capsaicin for use as a pesticide.

- The FDA does not require manufacturers to list all the food ingredients on a label. However, the new Food Allergen Labeling and Consumer Protection Act (S. 741), which becomes effective on January 1, 2006, requires labels to make clear which, if any, of the eight main food allergens—milk, eggs, peanuts, tree nuts, fish, crustacean shellfish, soy, and wheat—are present. The "hot" chili pepper is not included in this new legislation.

- Most food flavorings, natural flavorings, seasonings, spices, and spice extracts commonly used in foods as flavor enhancers or preservatives prior to the writing of the FDA food laws were not required to be proven safe after those laws became effective.

- The "hot" chili pepper is used in foods as a flavoring, a coloring, natural flavorings, a seasoning, a spice, or a spice extract.

7

A Primer on the "Hot" Chili Pepper and Toxic Capsaicin

The ingredients found to cause the most severe inflammation, pain, swelling, and stiffness in the food research group's investigations are present in the "hot" chili pepper, which belongs to the genus *Capsicum frutescens* of the Solanaceae plant family. Interestingly, the chili pepper is a cousin of the highly addictive tobacco plant, also a member of the Solanaceae family. Today people are aware of the severely harmful effects of tobacco. The Solanaceae family also includes the potato, the tomato, and the eggplant, which have been implicated in pain, swelling, and inflammation. Some of the participants in our studies, and a few whose experiences are documented in the Case Studies section of this book, found these other foods to be problematic also.

The "hot" chili pepper, a fruit that produces the "hot," peppery flavor in many common spicy dishes, is also in the spice known as cayenne pepper. That spice is made from the seeds and pods of capsicum peppers, which are of a species completely different from that of black pepper (*Piper nigrum*), a plant whose fruit is probably in the shaker on your table and was not found to be a problem food by our research group. The capsicum peppers are native to Mexico, Central America, the West Indies, and much of South America, but similar varieties are also native to the Far East. They may be long and thin like the cayenne pepper, large and firm like the Anaheim, cone shaped like the jalapeño, or small and cherry shaped. Peppers used to make a popular "hot" sauce are also of the genus *Capsicum frutescens*.

Ground red pepper, labeled "cayenne pepper" or simply "red pepper," is made of ground-up smaller, more pungent capsicums. The term "red pepper" may also be used to describe ground red pepper milder than cayenne. Crushed red pepper, the spice you find in pizza parlors, is made from the seeds of the "hot" varieties of *Capsicum annuum* and *Capsicum frutescens*. Chili powder is a blend of red pepper and other herbs and spices.

As I stated earlier, the chemicals that make peppers "hot" are the capsaicinoids (or alkaloids) concentrated in the pepper's seeds and membranes. Capsaicinoids are strong irritants that act directly on the pain receptors in your skin and mucous membranes. The strongest capsaicinoids are capsaicin and dihydrocapsaicin. Capsaicin is so strong that a single drop diluted in 1 million drops of water will warm your tongue. Like dihydrocapsaicin, it delivers a sting all over your mouth. A third capsaicinoid, nordihydrocapsaicin, produces a warmer, mellower sensation in the front of your mouth and on your palate. A fourth, homodihydrocapsaicin, packs a delayed punch, delivering a stinging, numbing burn to the back of your throat.

The irritant capsaicin, which when applied to the skin causes the small blood vessels under the skin to dilate, increases the flow of blood to the area and makes the skin feel warm. Hence it is used in popular topical medications that provide "pain relief," which contributes to people's general understanding of it as something beneficial.

But as capsaicin penetrates into the skin and muscles, it stimulates and then blocks local pain nerve fibers by completely depleting them of the neurotransmitter, "substance P." Substance P is the primary chemical messenger that relays pain to the brain. Initially, capsaicin causes the sensation of intense burning pain, followed by desensitization and the temporary relief of pain. *But there is no known resolution of the health problem that triggered the pain signal (such as inflammation of the muscle), even though the brain enjoys sensory relief.* Thus, you may "feel" better, but are you really better off?

To me, this situation resembles that of people inside a burning building who hear the fire alarm but can't see the source of the fire. Instead of finding the source of the fire and putting out the flames or escaping the burning building, they cut the wire to the fire alarm and put an end to the annoying alarm signal.

Capsaicin also stimulates nerve endings in your mouth and sends impulses to your brain that release endorphins, giving you a sense of well-being. The endorphin release might also explain the seemingly addictive quality of the plant. One individual I met, a man in his 20s whose hands were arthritic knots, kept a salt shaker filled with paprika on his kitchen table and liberally used the spice every day. He decided not to participate in one of our studies, because he could not bear to forgo this possible culprit in his diet. He said that eating paprika was one of his two pleasures. The other was smoking! I wonder how different this man's life might have been if he had been educated about food and pain when he was younger.

Information found in published pharmacological studies of the capsaicinoids shows that they produce a great variety of physiological responses affecting various bodily functions, such as strong irritation of the circulatory and respiratory reflexes, intensification of gastric peristalsis, stimulation of gastric acid production, inflammation and burning sensation of mucous membranes, and, in large doses, fatal hypothermia and symptoms similar to those of anaphylactic shock.

These ingredients also contribute to pain, swelling, and stiffness because they contain cholinesterase inhibitors that destroy the cholinesterase enzyme, which makes muscles move properly. The destruction of this enzyme causes pain, swelling, and muscle stiffness. In addition, these ingredients have now also been found to travel into the joints of test animals, where they affect the joint fluids and cause pain, stiffness, swelling, and accelerated wear and tear in cartilage. Eating "hot" chili peppers may also irritate the lining of your stomach or irritate your bladder so that you have to urinate more frequently. It could even make urination painful.

CHAPTER SEVEN RECAP

- The "hot" chili pepper belongs to the genus *Capsicum frutescens* of the Solanaceae plant family and is a cousin of the highly addictive, carcinogenic tobacco plant, also a member of the Solanaceae family.

- The "hot" chili pepper is also known as cayenne pepper, red pepper, and crushed red pepper.

- Capsaicin, the irritant in the "hot" chili pepper, acts on the pain receptors in the skin and mucous membranes, initially causing more pain followed by desensitization and interruption of the transmission of local pain signals to the brain.

- Capsaicin sends impulses to the brain that release endorphins, the body's "natural opiates," which create a temporary sense of well-being.

- Pharmacological studies show that capsaicin irritates the circulatory and respiratory reflexes, intensifies gastric peristalsis, stimulates gastric acid production, inflames mucous membranes, and in large doses can cause fatal hypothermia and symptoms similar to those of anaphylactic shock.

- Capsaicin contains cholinesterase inhibitors that destroy the cholinesterase enzyme, which makes muscles move properly. The destruction of this enzyme causes pain, swelling, and muscle stiffness.

8

How Much "Hot" Chili Pepper and Capsaicin Do Americans Eat?

According to the Chile Pepper Institute (www.chile pepperinstitute.org), the United States produces 885,630 metric tons, or 1,948,386,000 pounds, of "hot" chili pepper per year. Assuming we eat all that we produce, that's 2 billion pounds of "hot" chili pepper consumed per year in the United States. If we use 400,000,000 as a population figure, the 2 billion pounds that Americans consume translates into about five pounds of "hot" chili pepper per person, which includes men, women, *and children.*

Dr. Norman Childers, in his book *Arthritis—A Diet to Stop It,* says that the average capsaicin content of the "hot" chili pepper is 0.5 percent by weight of the whole pepper. This varies from 0.01 percent to up to 12 percent for the very hottest of the "hot" chili peppers.

If I multiply 0.5 percent (capsaicin in chili pepper) by 2,000,000,000 (number of pounds Americans consume annually), I get 10,000,000 pounds of capsaicin, or 0.025 pounds of capsaicin per person, equal to12 grams of capsaicin per person per year.

The book entitled *Sax's Dangerous Properties of Materials* lists the lethal oral dose of capsaicin as 47.2 mg/kg of body weight. According to this information, only two grams of capsaicin are needed to kill a 100-pound woman. *Only four grams of capsaicin are needed to kill a 200-pound man.*

The figures are dramatic and make a point. Could the number of grams of capsaicin consumed by Americans be lower? If we also assume that American food manufacturers export foods made with American "hot" chili pepper, that some of the food is consumed by people visiting from other countries, and that some is used as pesticide, then yes, the numbers would be lower. But even so, we know it takes only minute amounts of "hot" chili pepper to do harm.

Because of the Food and Health Research Group's investigations, I know that the "hot" chili pepper's capsaicin is in hundreds and possibly thousands of foods that Americans eat every day.

If we're consuming so much "hot" chili pepper, then, why aren't we all dropping dead from an overdose? From a toxicologist's point of view, the dose makes the poison: the greater the dose, the greater the effect on the body. Food manufacturers might argue that trace levels of the "hot" chili pepper's capsaicin used in food and found in the body do not pose a risk to health.

But then there's the question of what the cumulative effect of regularly eating capsaicin is. How does capsaicin interact with other natural toxins, like the nightshades tomato, potato, and eggplant? And what is the cumulative effect on people who eat chili pepper in combination with other foods that contain natural toxins?

Common popular foods like French-style salad dressing and pasta sauces are loaded with tomatoes and "hot" chili pepper. In the case of the dressing, the "hot" chili pepper is hidden in the vinegar in the recipe. Home fries, a common breakfast food, are made with potatoes and usually sprinkled with paprika, a food derived from "hot" chili pepper. These are just three "capsaicin cocktails" consumed by Americans every day.

As I stated earlier, some people seem not to have a problem when they eat "hot" chilies, but other people do. Maybe some of us are dropping dead from a variety of inflammation-related disorders, but at a lower, less obvious rate than if we ate a lethal dose in one sitting. *As far as I'm concerned, capsaicin was slowly killing me, and when I eliminated that toxin from my diet, I virtually eliminated the inflammation, pain, swelling, and stiffness I had endured for more than 50 years.*

CHAPTER EIGHT RECAP

- Two billion pounds of "hot" chili pepper are produced annually in the United States.

- *Sax's Dangerous Properties of Materials* lists the lethal oral dose of capsaicin as 47.2 mg/kg of body weight. According to this information, only two grams of capsaicin are needed to kill a 100-pound woman. Only four grams of capsaicin are needed to kill a 200-pound man.

- Questions to consider: What is the cumulative effect of the regular ingestion of capsaicin? How does capsaicin interact with other natural toxins, like those in the tomato, the potato, and the eggplant, which are also implicated in inflammation? And what is the cumulative effect on people who eat chili pepper in combination with other foods that have natural toxins?

9

Case Studies

I n the early '90s I organized the Arthritis Help Centers, a small group of professionals dedicated to helping people with arthritis by means of education and diet information. Over the years I have met or heard from hundreds of people who reduced or eliminated their inflammation, pain, swelling, and stiffness and improved their overall well-being by following the Arthritis Help Centers' dietary guidelines. The following individuals were happy to share their success stories. I hope they inspire you to consider taking a closer look at your diet and making positive changes.

GREG STROBEL, *head wrestling coach, Lehigh University, and U.S. Olympic wrestling coach*
"I'm sure I would have had my hip replaced years ago if I hadn't received help from the Arthritis Help Centers," says Greg Strobel, two-time coach for the U.S. Olympic wrestling team. Strobel, a competitive athlete for 12 years, has endured broken bones,

sprains, twisted ligaments, and aggravated joints. In his early 40s, despite the fact that his body is incredibly strong and resilient, he began to experience chronic pain.

Strobel ate "hot" red pepper every day. "I loved 'hot' peppers. I grew several exotic varieties in my backyard and made my own ground pepper and sauce so hot it would blister my mouth." Strobel is not arthritic, but he did have a degenerative right hip—the result, he believes, of repeated wrestling injuries as a youth. When his pain became chronic, he gave up running. "Walking only half a mile was excruciating. My hip ached so much I had trouble sleeping at all," says Strobel. The deterioration occurred while he was coaching the 1996 U.S. Olympic wrestling team.

"Meeting Ed Wendlocher and learning about his research was an eye opener for me," he says. As a coach, Strobel was well informed about nutrition and knew that food affects an athlete's performance. "But I was not aware of the alkaloid problem with some foods and that it could cause pain," he adds.

Making diet changes came easily for Strobel, who is very disciplined. "I simply stopped eating the 'hot' chili pepper," he states. "Within a month of changing my eating habits, I didn't need painkillers, and I haven't used them since. I could enjoy golf again because I wasn't in pain. I could even wrestle and demonstrate technique to my athletes." Strobel's regimen also included glucosamine chondroitin.

Strobel and his wife, who both love to cook, have adjusted their eating habits and are more conscious of the problem foods identified by the Arthritis Help Centers. "We cook for flavor now, not spiciness. I still make a great Kung Pow chicken!" He also shares his knowledge with his athletes. "They're young and skeptical. But I see the difference in their performance after Sunday night pepperoni pizza. On Monday, they're a little sluggish."

In 2000 Strobel coached the U.S. Olympic team in Sydney and was "basically pain-free as a result of following the advice on foods and taking health products." In the summer of 2003 Strobel had his right hip replaced, about four years later than he had intended. He continues to exercise five to six days a week.

TADD W., *information and knowledge management specialist*
Tadd W. woke up, got out of bed, and felt a pain like a hot iron stabbing at the back of his ankle. He was 20 years old and about to start the first semester of his junior year in college. That searing, unexpected early-morning incident unfolded into more than a decade of near-debilitating arthritis that traversed the lower half of his body and forever changed his life.

"I went to the doctor, sat outside his office surrounded by arthritic older people, and thought, 'This is what I have to look forward to—another 50 years of pain.'" Tadd's doctor diagnosed arthritis and put him on powerful drugs, including steroids. He was forced to give up tennis and soccer, the two sports he loved. His studies suffered. "I was in pain, and I had very little energy. My thinking became foggy. It was hard to maintain a positive outlook as I watched the physical activity I enjoyed taken away from me."

Today, at 38, Tadd skis, skates on Rollerblades, plays ice hockey, and rides his bike. In the summer of 2003 he hiked the Grand Canyon. "I'm especially proud of that hike," he says. Tadd attributes his recovery to his becoming educated about food and pain and changing his diet. "The Arthritis Help Centers helped me become conscious about what I eat. I completely avoid 'hot' chili peppers," he says. He is also scrupulous about reading food labels. "Problem foods are insidious. When I see the words *spices, artificial flavorings, natural flavorings,* or *colorings,* it's a red flag for me. I stay away." He also avoids canned condensed tomatoes.

Tadd first noticed that diet might be the cause of his problems when he returned from a 10-month career stint in Japan and the Philippines. "When I was away, I was nearly healed. When I came home, within three months I was sick again. That's when it dawned on me that something I was eating might be making me ill."

Shortly after returning home Tadd met a friend who was also having physical difficulties and was investigating food as a possible cause of his problems. This confirmed Tadd's suspicions and inspired him to experiment with "food avoidance." It was a frustrating period in his life, filled with trial and error, lacking support from the medical system, and even generating skepticism among fellow sufferers, whom he refers to as evincing "flat-earth syndrome."

"It is not a fallacy that what you eat affects your body. There's still resistance to the idea, but thank goodness that's changing. Look at all the press about low-carb dieting. This tells me that people are acknowledging that something besides fat might be contributing to national health problems. I hope to soon see elevated awareness about the relationship between certain foods and the painful symptoms of arthritis."

In 1995 Tadd met Professor John H. Abel, at Lehigh, who was conducting studies with the Arthritis Help Centers. After a long struggle, Tadd has been 95 percent pain-free for the past three years. "For the first time in years I feel as well as I did before the pain, swelling, and inflammation. I feel normal and in control of my life again. I'm completely off the arthritis medicine and only using two to six ibuprofen [pills] daily. My goal is to be off that, too. If I don't feel well, I believe it's because I've slipped off my diet and eaten something that's not good for me."

GAIL M., *real estate manager*
Gail M. was in her 50s when she sought help for pain in her joints. The first doctor she consulted advised her to wait and see how her condition progressed. Three years later, when her hands, wrists, elbows, and cheekbones were swollen and in pain, another doctor deemed her case hopeless and wanted to put her on medication immediately. "His waiting room was filled with people with walkers waiting for cortisone treatments. I knew that wasn't for me," she says.

Gail's story is unusual. Most doctors do not offer patients advice about nutrition and illness; witness the response of the first two she consulted. But her third physician, Dr. Leo Galland, whom she had consulted a decade earlier for colitis, told her that her condition might be related to food.

"After the 'death sentence' from my second doctor, I called Leo," she explains. "He asked me about my diet, particularly if I was eating 'hot' chili peppers. I told him that my boyfriend did most of the cooking and that he uses lots of chilies," she says.

Gail's boyfriend eliminated the "hot" pepper from their diet. "I immediately felt better. I was lucky. It was really that simple." Gail is vibrant and healthy and leads an active life, managing real estate, doting on her four grandchildren, and exercising regularly.

In 1995, when Dr. Galland first heard about Arthritis Help Centers from a patient of his who had found relief from inflammation and pain, he followed up with us and became a believer. Leo and I are still friends today. He recently shared with me the story of another patient who eradicated her inflammation when she eliminated the "hot" chili pepper from her diet. The case study is included in "A New Definition of Patient Centered Medicine," Dr. Galland's contribution to the professional text, *Integrated Medicine, A Systems Approach*, by Benjamin Kligler and Roberta Lee, McGraw Hill, New York, NY, 2004. I also recommend Dr. Galland's book, *The Four Pillars of Healing: How Integrated Medicine Can Heal You.*

JOSEPH K., *mechanical engineer, amateur mineralogist*
Joe K. has lived with rheumatoid arthritis for 15 years. Twelve of them have been pain-free. Joe was agile and moved freely well into his late 60s, when he began to experience pain that traveled between his hands, knees, elbows, and shoulders. Eventually the arthritis settled mostly in his hands. Driving a car became impossible, because he could not hold on to the steering wheel. The pain also interfered with his sleep. In addition, Joe's passion for miner-

alogy was dampened because he could not crack rocks open. The steroids, arthritis medication, and painkillers prescribed did not help him. Three years after being diagnosed, Joe heard about the Arthritis Help Centers' study at Lehigh University. "By then my pain was extreme, and I had to practically crawl to the school," says Joe.

As a participant in the study that included blood tests, Joe saw the dramatic difference in the blood samples taken before he ate possible problem foods and those taken afterward. Although he was still somewhat skeptical, he modified his diet and experimented with eliminating "hot" pepper, potato, tomato, and eggplant. He also took glucosamine sulfate. "I started to feel better. Within five months I was back in the quarry pounding rocks," he says.

Joe especially loves eggplant, one of the problem foods, and one day after his recovery from pain he decided to eat some. "Three days later, I was in agony. It was murder. Never again!" He also continues to avoid the "hot" pepper and the tomato. Potatoes do not seem to bother him. At 82 years of age, Joe is losing the flexibility in his hands. "But I have no pain from the arthritis, and I feel great." He continues to watch his diet, takes vitamin supplements, and has a very positive outlook on life.

Rosemary C., *artist and writer*

An artist and writer, Rosemary C. is sensitive, introspective, and contemplative by nature. She tends to view her life and physical health from a holistic perspective and is a proponent of the thinking that psychological, physiological, and environmental factors affect arthritis. "I don't think it's a coincidence that I was diagnosed with osteoarthritis of the knees shortly after my husband's untimely death. The shock and trauma of the loss were a burden that felt like too much to carry," she states. Rosemary did not arrive at her insight overnight. It's something she's been consciously exploring for a number of years in her writing and self-examination.

In tandem with her inner explorations, Rosemary investigated how diet influenced her condition. This approach was more appealing to her than taking arthritis medicine, which she says "did not sit well with [her] physically."

But when it was time to make a change in her diet, Rosemary resisted. "I had spent my whole life eating all the wonderful classic Italian meals I love, made with 'hot' red peppers and tomatoes," she says. She also admits she was a diet-cola "freak." Then, one day, within minutes of eating an eggplant parmigiana sandwich, she felt "an intense pain" in her knees, "like two giant toothaches." The pain convinced her of the correlation between food and pain and initiated her process of eliminating the problem foods identified in the Arthritis Help Centers' guidebook.

Today Rosemary says she no longer experiences the "deep, burning kind of pain" she recognizes as "food-related flare-up episodes." "My arthritis pain is mostly stress related, though I do feel it in high humidity or intense cold." Her daily regimen consists of taking one Aleve, one Tylenol, and vitamin supplements and of being aware of her diet.

LINDA L., *administrative assistant*

Linda was only 30 years old when she began to feel pain in her feet. It intensified until she had difficulty climbing three flights of stairs, as she had to do often during the workday. Linda was forced to find a new job when another company bought her employer. Fortunately, in her new position she no longer had to contend with the stairs. However, the inflammation and pain traveled to both hands—some friends say that one of her knuckles enlarged to the size of a golf ball. Eventually she was diagnosed with rheumatoid arthritis and began taking a variety of arthritis medications. Although she discussed diet with her doctors, they dismissed the nutritional approach without giving it much thought.

Linda heard about the Arthritis Help Centers' 100-person study hosted at Lehigh University and volunteered to be a participant. "I never would have put two plus two together in terms of my diet as a possible source of my pain," she states. Some of her favorite foods were tacos, salsa, pizza, and eggplant parmigiana.

"It was hard to eliminate the foods I like, but I began to notice that a few days after eating them I was in pain," she says. "I didn't expect the reaction to the wrong foods to occur two days later. Once I realized that, it was easier to determine which foods aggravated the disease." Linda explains that she still struggles with forgoing the "hot" pepper and tomatoes, "especially since we eat out a lot." A decade after being diagnosed with rheumatoid arthritis, she has significantly reduced her usage of medication and likes to imagine a day when she will need none.

Massachusetts General Hospital Reports Research That Confirms That Capsaicin Is a Potent Inflammatory Agent

I included the following press release, issued on September 25, 2002, by the Massachusetts General Hospital (www. massgeneral.com), because it addresses the connection between inflammation and pain and the "hot" chili pepper. It was posted on ScienceDaily.com on September 30, 2002. As of this writing, it resides in the archives of both websites.

ScienceDaily.com
09.03.02

CHILI PEPPERS AND INFLAMMATION: RESEARCHERS UNRAVEL MECHANISM OF PAIN SENSITIVITY

BOSTON—September 25, 2002. Scientists at Massachusetts General Hospital (MGH) have discovered a common component to the burning sensation produced by chili peppers and the pain associated with arthritis. The finding, published in the September 26 issue of *Neuron*, could help scientists devise new strategies to block the pain hypersensitivity associated with inflammation.

"The receptor activated by chili peppers in the mouth and other tissues also increases in the terminals of sensory neurons in the skin after inflammation, and this contributes to pain hypersensitivity," says Clifford Woolf, M.D., Ph.D., director of the Neural Plasticity Research Group in the Department of Anesthesia and Critical Care at MGH. A receptor is a protein that transports a chemical signal into a cell.

Woolf and lead author Ru-Rong Ji, Ph.D., also of the MGH Neural Plasticity Research Group, found that the increased production of the receptor following inflammation is mediated by a signal molecule called p38, located within sensory neurons. The chili pepper receptor, which is technically called TRPV1, responds to capsaicin, the chemical that is responsible for the "hot" in peppers. It also responds to actual heat and to low pH, a condition that occurs with inflammation.

"With these findings, we're starting to understand why patients with arthritis or other inflammatory conditions are likely to have increased pain and sensitivity to heat," says Woolf, who also is Richard J. Kitz Professor of Anaesthesia Research at Harvard Medical School. He and his research team were surprised to find that the activation of p38 can cause a twenty-fold increase in the amount of TRPV1 protein in the skin but not in the activity of the gene coding for TRPV1.

"This means that the chili pepper receptor is not being regulated by the gene being switched on but by more protein being produced, an unexpected form of regulation," says Ji. He also notes that their findings will open up new options for pain management. "We could use an inhibitor to p38 to block the increase in TRPV1, therefore blocking pain in patients who suffer from many diseases and conditions that involve inflammation."

Following inflammation, the activation of p38 is very precise. The scientists found that it is caused by a specific growth factor signal acting on a particular subset of pain sensory neurons. There are a variety of pain sensations that create different changes within neurons, and all of the signals that are generated have not yet been identified. Each new discovery, like the current finding by the MGH researchers, sheds light on these complex pathways and brings new treatment strategies closer.

The other members of the MGH research team are Tarek Samad, Ph.D., San-Xue Jin, Ph.D., and Raymond Schmoll, M.S., all of the MGH Neural Plasticity Research Group. The study was supported by grants from the National Institutes of Health.

Massachusetts General Hospital, established in 1811, is the original and largest teaching hospital of Harvard Medical School. The MGH conducts the largest hospital-based research program in the United States, with an annual research budget of more than $300 million and major research centers in AIDS, cardiovascular research, cancer, cutaneous biology, transplantation biology and photomedicine.

In 1994, the MGH joined with Brigham and Women's Hospital to form Partners HealthCare System, an integrated health care delivery system comprising the two academic medical centers, specialty and community hospitals, a network of physician groups, and nonacute and home health services.

CHAPTER TEN RECAP

- Scientists at the Massachusetts General Hospital (MGH) discovered a common component to the burning sensation produced by chili peppers and the pain associated with arthritis.

- Massachusetts General Hospital (MGH) reports research that confirms that capsaicin is a potent inflammatory agent.

- The receptor activated by chili peppers in the mouth and other tissues also increases in the terminals of sensory neurons in the skin after inflammation, and this contributes to pain hypersensitivity.

- The "chili pepper receptor," which is technically called TRPV1, responds to capsaicin, the chemical that is responsible for the "hot" in peppers.

11

The Solution, or,
"Doctor, It Hurts When I Do This"

found that the most effective way to reduce my inflammation and muscle and joint pain was to eliminate trigger foods from my diet. I recommend that you do so, too. Get them out of your kitchen. Avoid them at supermarkets, snack food stands, diners, and restaurants. Don't eat them.

I understand that the directive is easier said than followed. I remember when my cravings were so intense that I would get up at 2 a.m. and drive to the deli because I HAD to have potato salad made with red vinegar. That is the absolute truth.

Nobody wants to give up a food he loves. Diet is habitual, and food preferences are built over a lifetime. Young people are at a great advantage here, which is why I strongly advocate early education about good nutrition. They can develop healthy habits now that will last for a lifetime. *But all of us have the capacity to be aware of foods that might be harmful and the power to make the choice to avoid them.*

Because it was the "hot" chili pepper and its presence in spices, flavorings, and colorings that were found to be problematic, our recommendations are that you not eat the "hot" chili pepper in any form and that you eat a well-balanced diet, including foods from all the basic food groups. You need not feel deprived, for there are hundreds of wonderful foods to choose from.

My diet is filled with my favorite foods and has plenty of variety. Every meal is satisfying, and I'm never at a loss at a restaurant or a party. I am aware that some of my choices (bacon, red meat, sodas, sugar, and milk) are questionable among those who advocate the eating of only fresh fruit, vegetables, grains, and fish. Corn and wheat are also suspect. But through trial and error, I've discovered what works for me. *The one thing that is not beneficial for me, and for the hundreds of other people whom I've worked with or helped, is the "hot" chili pepper.*

When I go out to dinner, I remember my motto—**"Eat the spice, pay the price"**—and look forward to shrimp, crab, lobster, steak, chicken, or fish. I particularly enjoy Alfredo, Francese, and Marsala sauces. I might also have beer, plain wine, or plain liquor. If I want a soda, I'll choose Mountain Dew, Seven-Up, Sprite, or Sierra Mist.

I also eat a lot of fruit, including berries, apples, peaches, plums, cherries, and pears, which I grow on my farm. And I love chocolate!

A few words of caution about purchasing food from the supermarket and eating out. When you are shopping for food, read labels and check every ingredient. *Be especially careful when purchasing prepared foods, such as frozen dinners, canned meals, soups, sauces, dips, and condiments, many of which contain "hot" chili pepper spices.*

Today most restaurants' chefs accommodate special dietary requests. Talk to the wait staff; explain that you cannot eat certain foods, because they make you ill. Ask for help in selecting items that will not cause a problem. Tell them that you want your food to be as pure as possible. It's really not worth the several days of pain that will result if you eat a meal laced with the problem food ingredients!

CHAPTER ELEVEN RECAP

- THROW OUT problem foods! Right now, trash them.

- Enjoy a diet filled with lots of variety, including fresh fruit, vegetables, and protein.

- Read labels! Be wary of such terms as "flavoring," "coloring," "natural flavoring," "seasoning," "spice," and "spice extract."

- Be especially careful when purchasing prepared foods, such as frozen dinners, canned meals, soups, sauces, dips, and condiments, many of which contain "hot" chili pepper spices.

- Speak up at restaurants, and request food without paprika or other "hot" chili spices.

- Remember the Ed Wendlocher motto: "Eat the spice, pay the price!"

12

Inflammation Nation Impact Issues at a Glance

- The incidence of inflammatory disease is skyrocketing in the United States. Medical experts now link inflammation to heart attacks, heart disease, cancer, Alzheimer's, arthritis, and diabetes.

- Food consumption is directly related to inflammation and pain.

- The "hot" chili pepper, which contains capsaicin, a natural toxic food chemical, is an inflammatory food that is liberally used in a variety of forms in hundreds of prepared and processed foods.

- The "hot" chili pepper's capsaicin is highly toxic and has been approved as a pesticide by the Environmental Protection Agency. The EPA does not think it is necessary to test capsaicin for its effects on humans, because it is derived from the "hot" chili pepper, which is a commonly ingested food.

- Current food labeling laws do not require all ingredients to be listed on a food product label. A new law, which goes into effect January 1, 2006, has changed this for some foods (milk, eggs, fish, crustacean shellfish, tree nuts, peanuts, wheat, and soybeans), but not for the "hot" chili pepper. Some ingredients need be listed only as spices, flavorings, or colorings.

- The Food and Health Research Group, Inc., accurately identified, *for the first time,* ingredients in hundreds of foods and discovered that the "hot" chili pepper, which contains capsaicin, is present in those foods, though often hidden in the guise of spices, flavorings, or colorings.

- The Food and Research Group, Inc., and Arthritis Help Centers' participant studies demonstrated that the ingestion of foods containing the "hot" chili pepper consistently caused inflammatory episodes in some people and that the eliminating of foods containing the "hot" chili pepper consistently reduced inflammation and relieved pain in those people.

- Massachussets General Hospital (MGH) reports research that confirms that capsaicin is a potent inflammatory agent.

- Scientists at the Massachusetts General Hospital (MGH) discovered a common component to the burning sensation produced by chili peppers and the pain associated with arthritis. The receptor activated by chili peppers in the mouth and other tissues also increases in the terminals of sensory neurons in the skin after inflammation, and this contributes to pain hypersensitivity.

- "Eat the spice, pay the price!"

13

Food Lists: The Food and Health Research Group's Recommendations

The results of our food investigations are set forth in alphabetical order. First, you'll find the foods that contain the "hot" chili pepper, followed by a list of spices, herbs, and flavorings that we found not to be problematic. For your convenience, we've also created lists related to breakfast, lunch, dinner, desserts, beverages, and snacks. If there is a food you're curious about and it's not on any of our lists, write the Food and Health Research Group, Inc., at Box 768 Wharton, NJ 07885-0768 and we'll try to help you. Don't be dismayed by the list of foods that may be problematic for you. The list of recommended foods is much longer!

The Food and Health Research Group's Recommendations of Foods to Avoid and Foods Okay to Eat

Foods to Avoid

The primary food to avoid is the "hot" chili pepper, alone or in foods in any form: spices, flavorings, preservatives, or colorings.

Avoid the following:

allspice, balsamic vinegar, banana pepper, barbecue sauce, blackening, Bordelaise sauce, brown mustard, "Buffalo" sauces, Cajun spices, capsicum, catsup, cayenne pepper, chili pepper, chili powder, chili sauce, cocktail sauce, cole slaw, Creole cooking, cumin, curry powder, deviled foods, Dijon mustard, five-spice powder, flavorings made from spices, gravies, "hot" pepper, "hot" sauce, Hunan spices, ketchup, mace, marinades, marinara sauce, mayonnaise, mustard, "natural flavorings" made from spices, oleoresin paprika, paprika, pepper (cayenne), pepper (chili), pepper (red "hot"), pepper (white), pickles, pickled foods, pizza sauce (red), poultry seasoning, ranch dressing, red-hots, red pepper, red vinegar, salad dressings, salsa, salt substitutes (spicy), sautéed foods, scampi sauce, seasonings, Sichuan spices, soup bases, spices, spicy dips, spice extracts, spiced vinegar, steak sauces, Tex-Mex spices, Thai spices, tomato concentrates, tomato sauces, Vietnamese spices, vinaigrette dressing, vinegar (red), vinegar (spiced), vinegar (wine), white pepper, wine vinegar, Worcestershire sauce, yellow mustard.

The following popular food items require special attention, as the problem food ingredients are often hidden:

bread crumbs (many kinds), canned tuna (most), catsup, coated peanuts (some), deli meats and salads (most), home fries (some), ketchup, mayonnaise (some), Muenster cheese (rind), pickles (most), pizza (most, white pizza is okay), prepared entrées (most), prepared gravies (most), prepared pies (some), prepared salad dressings (most), prepared sauces (most), prepared soups (most), red wine vinegar, restaurant seafood (most; often sprinkled with paprika).

Foods Okay to Eat

It's okay to eat the following herbs, spices, and flavorings:
anise, amandine style, annatto, apple cider vinegar, artificial sweeteners, aspartame, baking powder, balm, bay leaf, basil, black pepper, brown sugar, butter, cane sugar, capers, caraway, cardamom, celery seed, chamomile, cherry, chicory, chives, chocolate, cilantro, cinnamon, citrus, cloves, coriander, cream of tartar, dandelion, dill, fennel, fenugreek, Français sauce or style, fruit flavorings, garlic, ginger, green pepper, honey, hops, horseradish (plain), Italian parsley, lavender, lemon, licorice, lime, lovage, margarine, marjoram, Marsala sauce, marshmallow, natural flavorings from fruits, nondairy creamers, nutmeg, olive oil, onions, orange, oregano, parsley, pepper (black), pepper (green sweet), pepper (red sweet), peppercorns, peppermint, pine nuts, pizza sauce (white), poppy seeds, raspberry, rose hips, rosemary, saccharin, saffron, sage, salt, savory, scallions, sesame, shallots, smoked foods, sorrel, sour cream, soy sauce, spearmint, sugar, sweet pepper, sweet cicely, tarragon, thyme, turmeric, vanilla, vegetable oils, vinegar (apple cider), vinegar (white), watercress.

Common Meals, with Foods to Avoid and Foods Okay to Eat

Breakfast

Avoid the following:
Canadian-style bacon, ham (spiced), home fries with paprika, sausage, spiced ham, tomato juice, vegetable drinks.

Okay to eat the following:

apple juice, bacon (American), bagel (plain), berries, bread, butter, cantaloupe, cereals, citrus, coffee, corn muffin, cranberry juice, cream, croissant, Danish, doughnut, eggs, egg substitute, farina, French toast, fruit, grapefruit, ham, home fries, honeydew melon, instant breakfast, jam, jelly, maple syrup, margarine, melon, milk, muffin, oatmeal, orange juice, pancakes, preserves, prune juice, rolls, rye bread, sugar, sugar substitutes, syrup, tea, toast, waffles.

Lunch/Dinner

Avoid the following:

antipasti, baked beans (spicy), balsamic vinegar, barbecue sauce, bean salad*, blackened foods, bologna, Buffalo wings, burritos, canned soups*, Cajun foods, casseroles*, catsup, cayenne pepper, chicken salad*, chicken soup*, chili, Chinese foods (spicy), cole slaw, curried foods, deviled foods, cream sauces (with spices), dried soup mixes, eggplant, fajitas, fish (breaded with spices in bread crumbs), fish (with paprika), frankfurters, gravies, ham (spiced), hot dogs, "hot" sauces, "hot" pepper, Hunan style, jalapeño peppers, ketchup, kielbasa, lasagne*, liverwurst, macaroni salad*, manicotti*, marinades, mayonnaise, meat sauces (spicy), Mexican style, minestrone soup, Muenster cheese, mustard, nachos, nuggets (with spiced crumbs), onion soup, Oriental style (spicy), pasta salads*, pasta sauces, peanut butter*, pickles, pickled foods, pizza (red), potato salad, ravioli, red sauces, red pepper, red vinegar, relishes, roasted pepper, salad dressings*, salsa, salt substitutes, sausages, sautéed foods*, seasonings, shrimp salad*, Sichuan style, soups*, spicy foods, steak (marinade), stews, stuffing*, tacos, tamales, teriyaki, Tex-Mex foods, Thai foods (spicy), tomato concentrates, tomato sauces, tuna (with vegetable broth), vegetable soup, Vietnamese foods (spicy), vinaigrettes, wine vinegar.

* Often made with paprika or other forms of "hot" chili pepper.

Okay to eat the following:
American cheese, apple cider vinegar, asparagus, basil, beans, beef, biscuits, black pepper (the one in the shaker), bread, broccoli, broth, burger, cabbage, carrots, cauliflower, clams, cream cheese, celery, cheddar cheese, cheeseburger, chicken, chicken Français, chives, clams, corn, cottage cheese, crab, crackers, cranberry, cream sauces, croissants, cucumber, dill, dumplings, egg roll, fettuccine Alfredo, fish, fish Français, French fries (plain), garlic, green beans, greens, ham, hamburger, lamb, lemon juice, lettuce, lima beans, liver, lobster, Monterey Jack cheese, mozzarella cheese, mussels, noodles, noodles Parmesan, olive oil, onion, oregano, Parmesan cheese, pasta (plain), peas, pepper (black), pita bread, pizza (white), pork, potato, rice, rye bread, salad, salmon, salt, shallots, shellfish, shrimp, snow peas, sour cream, spaghetti (pasta), spinach, squash, steak, sweet potato, Swiss cheese, ricotta cheese, tomato, tuna (without vegetable broth), turkey, veal, veal Français, vegetable oil, wax beans, white vinegar, yogurt.

Snacks and Desserts

Avoid the following:
spicy snacks or desserts.

Okay to eat the following:
apple, apple crisp, applesauce, almonds, bananas, berries, brownies, butterscotch, cake, candy, carrots, cashews, celery, crackers (plain), cheesecake, cherries, chocolate, cookies, custard, doughnuts, fruit pies, fruits, fudge, gelatin, grapes, ice cream, ice milk, melon, milk chocolate, nuts, oranges, peaches, peanuts, pears, pecans, pineapple, pistachios, plums, popcorn, potato chips (not spicy), pretzels, pudding, raisins, strawberries, walnuts, watermelon, whipped cream, yogurt.

Drinks

Avoid the following:

colas (yes, some colas, including major brands, are made with red pepper), pepper drinks, root beer, rum (spiced), spicy drinks, tea (spiced herbal), vegetable drinks, whiskey (spiced), wine (spiced).

Okay to drink the following:

beer, champagne, chocolate drinks, club soda, coffee, fruit juices, grape juice, hot chocolate, iced coffee, iced tea, lemonade, lemon/lime, milk, milk shake, Mountain Dew®, orange juice, orangeade, orange soda, rum, Seven-Up®, shakes, Sierra Mist®, Snapple® fruit drinks, Sprite®, tea, vodka, water, whiskey, wine.

The Food and Health Research Group's Recommended Foods, Listed Alphabetically

Remember to always check for added spices and flavorings.

A

abalone

acorn squash

albacore tuna

alcohol

alcohol-free beer

ale

alfalfa

Alfredo sauce

all-purpose flour

almond

amandine style

ambrosia dessert

American cheese

anchovy

angelfish

angel food cake

anise

Anjou pear

annatto

apple

apple butter

apple cider vinegar

apple crisp

apple fritter

applejack

applesauce

apricot

artificial sweeteners

artichoke

artichoke (Jerusalem)

artichoke hearts

arugula

asparagus

aspartame

au gratin style

avocado

B

bacon (American)

bacon bits

bagel
baked Alaska
baked beans
   (plain)
baked ham
baked potato
baking powder
baking soda
bamboo shoots
banana
banana bread
banana cream pie
banana split
barley
Bartlett pear
basil
Bavarian cream
bay leaf
beans (dried)
beans (green)
beans (lima)
bean sprouts
beef
beef burger
beef roast
beef short ribs
beer
beet
beet greens
Belgian endive
Belgian waffle
bell pepper (sweet)
Bermuda onion
Bibb lettuce

Bing cherry
birch beer
biscuit
bittersweet
   chocolate
black bean
blackberry
black cherry
black coffee
black currant
black-eyed peas
black olives
black pepper
black walnut
blended oils
blended whiskey
blintz
blowfish
blueberry
blue cheese
bluefish
blush wine
boiled ham
bock beer
boilermaker
bok choy
Bosc pear
Boston cream pie
Boston lettuce
bottom round
bourbon
bow tie pasta
boysenberry
bran

bran cereals
brandy
Brazil nut
bread
bread crumbs
   (plain)
bread flour
breading
bread pudding
brick cheese
Brie cheese
brine
broadleaf lettuce
broccoli
broccoli rab
brown bread
brownie
brown mushroom
brown rice
brown sugar
Brussels sprouts
brut
bubble gum
buckwheat
bun
bunching onions
burger
burger and fries
burrito (plain)
butter
buttercup squash
butterfish
butter flavoring
butterhead lettuce

butter/margarine
   blends
buttermilk
butternut squash
butter sauce
butterscotch
butter substitutes

C

cabbage
Cabernet
cacao
caffeine
cake
cake flour
calamari
chamomile
candy apple
candied fruit
canned ham (plain)
canola oil
cantaloupe
capers
capon
cappuccino
caramel
caramel custard
caraway
carbonated water
cardamom
carob
carob bean gum
carp
carrageen

carrot
carrot sticks
cashew
catfish
cauliflower
caviar
chef salad
celeriac
celery
celery salt
celery seed
celtuce
cereal grains
Champagne
Champagne
   cocktail
chard
cheddar cheese
cheese balls
cheesecake
cheese food
cherries jubilee
cherry
cherrystone clams
cherry tomato
chestnuts
chewing gum
chicken
chicken Francese
chicken livers
chickpeas
chicory
chicory coffee
chiffon cake

chiffon pie
Chinese cabbage
Chinese chard
Chinese chestnut
Chinese egg noodle
chives
chocolate
chocolate chip
   cookies
chocolate chips
chocolate fudge
chocolate milk
chocolate syrup
chuck beef
cider
cider vinegar
cinnamon
citric acid
citrus fruit
clam
clam juice
clementines
cling peach
clove
club soda
club steak
cobbler
cocktail
cocktail nuts
cocktail peanuts
cocoa
cocoa butter
cocoa powder
coconut

codfish
cod liver oil
coffee
coffee creamers
Cognac
Colby cheese
Cold Duck
collard greens
colored sugar
comb honey
conch
Concord grape
condensed milk
confectioners' sugar
consommé
converted rice
cooking oils
cooking sprays
cooking wines
coon cheese
coriander
corn
corn bread
corn cakes
corn cereals
corn chips
corn flakes
corn flour
Cornish game hen
cornmeal
corn oil
corn on the cob
corn pudding
cornstarch

corn syrup
corn tortilla (plain)
corn whiskey
Cos lettuce
cottage cheese
cottage fries
cotton candy
cottonseed oil
cowpeas
crab
crab apple
cracked wheat
crackers
cranberry
cranberry sauce
crayfish
cream
cream cheese
cream filled
   doughnut
creamed corn
creamery butter
Cream of Wheat
cream puffs
cream pie
Crenshaw melon
crêpe
cress
croissant
crookneck squash
croutons
cruller
cucumber
cupcake

curly parsley
currant
custard dessert
custard pie

D
daikon lettuce
daiquiri
dandelion
dates
decaffeinated coffee
dessert toppings
dessert wines
devil's food cake
diet Seven-Up
diet margarine
diet Sprite
dill
dinner wine
distilled vinegar
distilled water
dough
doughnut
Dover sole
draft beer
dried beef
dry milk
dry-roasted nuts
duck
dumplings
durum wheat
Dutch-process
   cocoa

E

éclair
Edam cheese
eel
eggnog
egg noodles
eggs
egg substitute
elderberries
elephant garlic
endive
English muffins
English walnuts
enriched white
    bread
enzymes
escargot
espresso
evaporated milk
extra-virgin olive
    oil

F

farina
fats
fava bean
fennel
fennel seed
fenugreek
feta cheese
fettuccine
fettuccine Alfredo
fiber
filberts

Fig Newtons
figs
filet
filet mignon
fish
fish and chips
fish sticks
flambé style
flan
flapjacks
flounder
flour (potato)
flour (rye)
flour (wheat)
fondue
fortune cookie
Francese sauce
freestone peaches
French bread
French Colombard
French fries
French toast
fried chicken
frogs' legs
frostings
frozen yogurt
fructose
fruitcake
fruit candy
fruit cocktail
fruit juices
fruit-flavored syrup
fruit flavorings
fruits

fruit salad
fudge
fudge cookies
Fuji apple
funnel cake

G

Gamay wine
game meat
garbanzo beans
garden peas
garlic
Gatorade
gelatin
gelatin desserts
ginger
ginger ale
gingerbread
gingersnaps
glaze
glucose
gluten
goose
gooseberry
Gouda cheese
Graham crackers
Graham flour
grains
Granny Smith
    apple
granola
granola bars
grapefruit
grape leaves

grapes
grease
green beans
green olives
green onion
green peas
green pepper
　(sweet)
greens
Grenache wine
grenadine
griddle cakes
grits
ground beef
grouper fish
grouse
guava
gum
gum arabic
gumbo
gumdrops

H
haddock
half-and-half
halibut
ham
hamburger
Hamburg parsley
hamburger steak
hake
hard-boiled egg
hard candies
hard cider

hard roll
hard-shell clam
hash brown
　potatoes
hazelnut
head lettuce
heart of palm
heavy whipping
　cream
herring
hickory-smoked
　flavor
highball
hoagie roll
home-fried
　potatoes (plain)
hominy
homogenized milk
honey
honeydew melon
hops
horehound candy
horseradish
hot chocolate
hot cross bun
hot fudge
Hubbard squash
hydrogenated oils
hydrolyzed
　vegetable protein

I
iceberg lettuce
ice cream

iced tea
iced tea with lemon
ice milk
icicle radish
icing
instant coffee
instant mashed
　potatoes
instant tea
invert sugar
iodized salt
Irish coffee
Irish soda bread
iron
Italian bread
Italian green beans
Italian ices
Italian parsley

J
jams
jasmine tea
Java
jelly
jelly beans
jelly rolls
Jerusalem artichoke
juice (apple)
juice (fruit)
juice (orange)

K
kaiser roll
kale

kelp
Key lime pie
kidneys
king crab
kiwifruit
kohlrabi
kumquat

L

lactose
ladyfingers
lager beer
lamb
lamb chops
lard
lavender
leaf lettuce
lecithin
leek
legumes
lemon
lemonade
lemon balm
lemon/lime
lemon meringue
  pie
lemon soda
lemon thyme
lettuce
licorice
light cream
lime
lingonberry
linguine

liquors
littleneck clams
liver
lobster
locust bean gum
London broil
long-grain rice
longhorn cheese
low-calorie
  sweeteners
low-fat milk
lox (plain)

M

Macadamia nuts
macaroni
macaroni and
  cheese
macaroon
mackerel
maize
malt
malt liquor
malted milk
mandarin orange
mango
maple syrup
maraschino cherry
margarine
marjoram
marmalade
marshmallow
Marsala wine
martini

mashed potato
matzo
matzo balls
Macintosh apple
meats
meatballs
meat tenderizer
Melba toast
melon
menthol
meringue
milk
milk chocolate
milk shake
millet
mineral water
mint candy
mint leaf
mixed grill
mixed nuts
mocha
molasses
mollusk
monosodium
  glutamate
Monterey Jack
  cheese
Mountain Dew®
  soda
mousse
mozzarella cheese
Mueslix
muffin
mulberry

mullet
mung bean
mushrooms
muskmelon
mussels
mustard greens
mustard seed
mutton

N
nachos (plain)
Napoleons
navel orange
navy beans
nectarine
new potato
nondairy creamers
nonfat milk
noodles
nougat
nuts
nutmeg

O
oat cereals
oat flour
oatmeal
oats
octopus
oil (corn)
oil (cottonseed)
oil (olive)
oil (palm)
oil (peanut)

okra
oleomargarine
olive oil
olives
omelets
onion powder
onions
orange
orangeade
orange juice
orange peel
orange soda
oregano
oxtail
oyster crackers
oysters

P
pak choi
palm hearts
palm oil
pancakes
papaya
parfait
Parmesan cheese
parsley
parsnips
passion fruit
pasta
pattypan squash
peaches
peach brandy
peach Melba
peanut brittle

peanut butter
   (fresh)
peanut oil
peanuts
pear
pearl onions
peas
pecan pie
pecans
pectin
pepper (black)
pepper
   (green sweet)
pepper (red sweet)
peppercorns
peppermint
persimmon
pheasant
phyllo
piecrust
pignolia nuts
pigs' feet
pimiento (sweet)
piña colada
pineapple
pine nuts
pink beans
pink grapefruit
pinto bean
pistachio nuts
pita bread
pizza (white)
plums
plum tomato

polysorbate
pomegranate
popcorn
Popsicles
poppy seeds
pork
potato
potato bread
potato chips
potato flour
potato pancakes
poultry
pound cake
powdered milk
powdered soft-
    drink mixes
pralines
prawns
preserves
pretzels
provolone cheese
prune butter
prunes
pudding desserts
puffed rice
puffed wheat
pumpernickel
    bread
pumpkin
punch

Q
quail

R
rabbit
radicchio
radish
raisin bran cereals
raisins
rapeseed
raspberry
red cabbage
red potato
red snapper
rennet
rhubarb
riboflavin
ribs
rice
rice cakes
rice cereals
rice flour
rice pudding
ricotta cheese
ripe olives
Rock Cornish hen
rock lobster
roe
roll
rolled oats
roma bean
romaine
Romano cheese
Roquefort cheese
rosé wine
rosemary
rum

Russian caviar
rutabaga
rye bread
rye flour
rye whiskey

S
saccharin
safflower oil
saffron
sage
salads
salmon
salsify
salt
saltines
saltwater taffy
sardines
sarsaparilla
sauerkraut
savory
Savoy cabbage
scallions
scalloped potatoes
scallops
scrambled eggs
Scotch
scrod
seafood (plain)
seaweed
seedless grapes
seltzer water
semisweet
    chocolate

semolina
sesame seed
7-Up® soda
shakes
shallots
shark
shellfish
shell pasta
sherbet
sherry
shoestring potato
shoofly pie
shortbread
shortcake
shortening
shredded wheat
shrimp
Sierra Mist® soda
sirloin
skim milk
Slice soda
smoked cheese
smoked foods
smoke flavor
snail
snap peas
snapper
Snapple® fruit
    drinks
snow cones
snow peas
soda crackers
soft-shell crab
sole

sorbet
sorbitol
sorghum
soufflé
sour cream
sourdough
sour milk
soybean
soy protein
spaghetti pasta
spaghetti squash
Spanish onion
Spanish peanut
spareribs (plain)
sparkling wines
spearmint
spinach
Sprite® soda
squab
squash
squid
starch
steak
steak fries
steak tartare
steamer clams
sticky bun
string beans
strawberries
streusel cake
strudel
succotash
sucrose
sugar

sugar snap peas
sugar substitutes
sundaes
sunflower seeds
sun tea
surf 'n' turf
sushi
sweet butter
sweet chocolate
sweet cider
sweet corn
sweet marjoram
sweet pepper
sweet potato
Swiss chard
Swiss cheese
Swiss-style yogurt
swordfish
syrup

T

table salt
taco (plain)
taffy
tangelo
tangerine
tapioca
tarragon
tea
tenderizer
tenderloin
tequila
thyme
toast

toffee
tofu
tomato (fresh)
tongue
tonic
torte
tortellini
tortilla
tossed salad
tripe
trout
truffles
tuna (without
    vegetable broth)
turban squash
turkey
turmeric
turnip greens
turnips

U
ultrapasteurized
    milk
unsalted butter

V
vanilla

vanillin
veal
veal Francese
vegetable oil
vegetable protein
venison
vermicelli
Vermont cheddar
vermouth
Vidalia onion
vinegar (apple
    cider)
vinegar (white)
vitamin A, B's, C, D,
    and E
vodka (grain)

W
waffle
walnuts
watercress
watermelon
wax bean
wheat
whey
whiskey
white beans

whitefish
white pizza
white sauces
white sugar
whole grains
whole wheat
whipped cream
wild rice (plain)
wine
wine cooler
Winesap apple
wintergreen
winter squash

Y
yams
yard-long bean
yeast
yellow wax bean
yogurt
yuca

Z
ziti pasta
zucchini

14

What Else Can Be Done?

In addition to eliminating the "hot" chili pepper, in any form, from your diet, we recommend the following tactics:

1. Tell your friends, family, and physician about the potent inflammatory, toxic pesticide capsaicin in food.

2. Contact federal, state, and local food safety agencies and ask them, "Why is the potent inflammatory, toxic pesticide capsaicin allowed in the foods we eat every day without safety testing?"

3. Notify federal, state, and local elected officials about this food safety problem and the lack of accurate food labeling of capsaicin.

4. Contact food manufacturers and let them know you want capsaicin identified on a label if it is in the food.

Addendum

Additional Research Conducted by the Arthritis Help Centers

In 1995 Drs. Abel and Nau conducted a 100-person study for the Arthritis Help Centers. After additional food ingredient investigations were completed, the 100-person study was planned to evaluate whether persons with arthritis could benefit both by not eating the foods found to cause pain, swelling, and stiffness and by taking specially formulated health products. The health products to be included were selected as the most effective of the many available at the time during a prescreening process. This study included more than 100 persons suffering from one or more types of arthritis at various levels of severity of pain, swelling, and stiffness. The most common types of arthritis among persons in the studies were osteoarthritis and rheumatoid arthritis. This study was scientifically designed and included a carefully monitored, two-month double-blind study with a placebo control group.

100-person prestudy

Professor John Abel, Ph.D., Eugene Nau, Ph.D., Roman Bielski, Ph.D., and I carefully designed the 100-person study. We also had assistance from local practicing rheumatologists.

Persons afflicted with arthritis were invited to participate through numerous ads placed in local newspapers. Approximately 150 individuals called and offered to participate. Those persons were invited to a group meeting on a Sunday evening at Iacocca Hall at Lehigh University, in Bethlehem, Pennsylvania. I gave a background presentation and an explanation of the study. Eugene Nau, Ph.D., explained the study objectives. Three graduate students were on hand to help answer individual questions, to distribute study information packages, and to request signatures on a sign-up sheet.

More than 100 persons signed up and received the study information packages. These packages included start-up instructions, an informed consent form, a patient questionnaire, an activities and lifestyle index, a pain index, a joint structure form, and a tender joint count, to be completed at the start of the study. The patient questionnaire recorded basic information about the patient. The activities and lifestyle index ranked nine common activities at the beginning of the study and at its end. The pain index form enabled each individual to record his or her perception of pain at the beginning of the study and at its end. The joint structure sheet allowed each individual to complete an appraisal of joint condition at the beginning of the study and at the end. The tender joint count gave each individual the opportunity to provide an appraisal of his or her joint pain at the beginning of the study and at the end.

The Study

Each participant was scheduled in turn to visit the university to start the study. Dr. Nau, medically qualified assistants, and graduate student assistants were there to process each participant. A study package was distributed to and reviewed with each participant, an ID number was assigned, a numbered package of health products or a placebo was distributed, grip strength was measured and recorded, and blood samples were taken from each participant.

Each individual recorded the foods eaten each day and recorded his or her daily condition in a daily condition assessment journal. Each participant was scheduled in turn to visit the university at the end of the study. Dr. Nau, medically qualified assistants, and graduate student assistants were on hand to process each participant. The study package was received back and reviewed with each participant, grip strength was measured and recorded, and blood samples were again taken from each participant. Blood tests taken included (1) immune complexes (the relative amount of immune complexes were measured at the beginning of the study and at the end using a specially developed ELISA); (2) cortisol (the levels of cortisol were measured at the beginning of the study and at the end); and (3) erythrocyte sedimentation rate (ESR) (the ESR levels were measured at the beginning of the study and at the end).

The Results

The results of this study clearly showed that pain intensity increased *severely* for many patients starting one to two days after they ate certain foods. Seventy-eight percent (78%) of the participants who did not eat the problem foods and took specially formulated health products showed significant improvement in their arthritic condition. Pain was measured by a comparison between the patient's ranking of pain recorded before the study and that recorded following the study. **Pain was reported as reduced by an *average* of 34 percent for the group not eating any problem foods and taking the health products.** Inflammation was measured by a comparison of blood tests of immune complexes recorded before the study with those recorded following the study. **Inflammation was measured as reduced by an average of 29 percent for the group not eating the problem foods and taking the health products.**

Observations

Most persons in the study experienced a seven-day cycle for each problem food ingredient eaten. Consider Day 1 as the day the problem food ingredient is eaten. Many experienced symptoms as follows:

DAY 1—Increased body temperature and thirst.

DAY 2—General poor feeling with continued increased body temperature and thirst. Some pain, stiffness, swelling, and impaired ability in the affected joints and muscles (usually the joints and muscles used the most).

DAY 3—Severely increased pain, stiffness, swelling, and impaired ability in the affected joints and muscles.

DAY 4—Continued severely increased pain, stiffness, swelling, and impaired ability in the affected joints and muscles.

DAY 5—Decrease in pain, stiffness, swelling, and impaired ability.

DAY 6—Significantly decreased pain, stiffness, swelling, and impaired ability.

DAY 7—No apparent continued effect of the problem food ingredient eaten on Day 1.

ADDENDUM RECAP

- **In a 100-person study designed to evaluate whether persons with arthritis could benefit both by not eating the foods found to cause pain, swelling, and stiffness and by taking specially formulated health products, the results clearly showed that pain intensity in-**

creased severely for many patients starting one to two days after they ate certain foods.

- Seventy-eight percent (78%) of the participants who did not eat the problem foods and took specially formulated health products showed significant improvement in their arthritic condition.

- Pain was reported reduced by an average of 34 percent for the group not eating any problem foods and taking the health products.

- Inflammation was measured as being reduced by an average of 29 percent for the group not eating the problem foods and taking the health products.

- Most persons in the study experienced a seven-day cycle with each problem food ingredient eaten.

Bibliography

The Code of Federal Regulations. National Archives and Records Administration, Washington, D.C.

The Complete Book of Herbs, Spices and Condiments. Carol Ann Rinzler. Facts On File, Inc., New York, N.Y.

The Complete Book of Spices. Jill Norman. Penguin Books, New York, N.Y.

The Cook's Encyclopedia. Tom Stobart. Harper & Row Publishers, New York, N.Y

The Dictionary of American Food and Drink. John Mariani. Hearst Books, New York, N.Y.

The Food Chronology. James Trager. Henry Holt & Co., New York, N.Y.

Joy of Cooking. Irma S. Rombauer, Marion Rombauer Becker, and Ethan Becker. Scribner, New York, N.Y.

Modern Nutrition in Health and Disease. Alfred Jay Bollet. Lea & Febiger, Philadelphia, Pa.

The Nightshades and Health. Norman F. Childers and Gerard M. Russo. Somerset Press, Inc., Somerville, N.J.

Sax's Dangerous Properties of Materials. Richard J. Lewis Sr. John Wiley & Sons, Inc., New York, N.Y.

The Scientist, October 14, 2002, v. 16, i. 20, p. 8 (1). "Hot research, burning pain: the protein TRPV is sensitive to capsaicin, found in chili peppers."

ScienceDaily.com, September 30, 2002. "Chili Peppers and Inflammation: Researchers Unravel Mechanism of Pain Sensitivity."

They All Laughed at Christopher Columbus. Gerald Weissmann, M.D. Time Books, New York, N.Y.

Time, December 9, 2002. "The Age of Arthritis. We're headed for an epidemic of joint disease. What you can do to protect yourself."

Time, February 23, 2004. "The Secret Killer. The surprising link between inflammation and heart attacks, cancer, Alzheimer's and other diseases. What you can do to fight it."

Casarett and Doull's *Toxicology*. McGraw-Hill, New York, N.Y.

ABOUT THE COAUTHOR

Claudia Kreiss is a public relations professional, writer, yoga instructor, and artist. Contact her at *claudiakreiss@att.net.*